Intermittent Fasting for Women

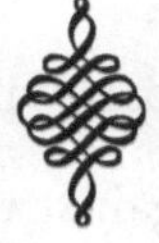

Hidden Truths About Losing Weight and Living a Healthy Life Effortlessly

By

Jamie Knight

purposes only. All effort has been executed to present accurate, up to date, and reliable, complete information. No warranties of any kind are declared or implied. Readers acknowledge that the author is not engaging in the rendering of legal, financial, medical or professional advice. The content within this book has been derived from various sources. Please consult a licensed professional before attempting any techniques outlined in this book.

By reading this document, the reader agrees that under no circumstances are is the author responsible for any losses, direct or indirect, which are incurred as a result of the use of information contained within this document, including, but not limited to, —errors, omissions, or inaccuracies.

Table of Contents

Introduction

The longest I've fasted is thirty days. I lost thirty pounds, altered my eating habits, changed my mood, and I fitted into smaller clothes. For the first five days, it was the hardest thing I had ever done. The rest of the time, for twenty-five days, there were easy days, and there were hard days. The hard days, however, became progressively easier.

It turns out that it's not the lack of food that stresses your body. It is the breaking of a habit (the habit of eating regular meals) that tortures your mind.

Don't worry. Fasting for thirty days is not a prerequisite for intermittent fasting. I just wanted to share with you where I am coming from. When you fast for thirty days straight, without any food, subsisting only on water, the body heals itself, from scars and loose skin on the outside, to cysts and imbalances on the inside. Even irregular menstrual cycles tend to get in line.

I just completed a thirty-day fast in April, and everything from my joint pains on cold mornings, to my varying levels of anxiety, came to a gentle halt. I've read first-person experiences of things like tumors that shrink and get digested by the body; I didn't have any tumors so I can't attest to that, but I can tell you that my persistently blocked nose (from acute allergies) are gone and my need for a daily dose (sometimes two) of antihistamines are also a thing of the past.

Toxins that accumulate in the fatty tissue within the flesh are flushed out along with the fat that is burned; the mind realigns to what millions of years of nature's evolution has endowed it with; and the burden of an imbalanced existence is cast off in exchange for the energy and calm of the wise.

The 30-day fast is a far cry from the Intermittent Fast (IF) in terms of the intensity of it all, but I have found that the effects and benefits are almost identical without the initial onset of discomfort. You can think of IF as a more efficient method of getting the same results.

Most people aren't geared to do 30-day fasts. We have schedules and obligations that will hinder and disrupt it. It is, however, easily integrated into any schedule and gives you about 70% of the results that the full 30-day fast will give you. That's a good deal.

As we unfold the methods and practices of intermittent fasting, we will unveil the differences in the two and how you can take it easy with IF or you can supercharge it. The intensity is up to you, on the proviso that you reach the minimum threshold which will alter the way the body's physiology changes.

There are ten things you need to know about the relationship between the human body and the food we eat. Once you get a good understanding of this platform, you will get a good idea of why, if, or any other kinds of fasting for that matter does the body good.

1. The main function of food is to provide energy and nutrients to the body.

2. Taste is not just about pleasure; it's about identifying the nutrients that we need.

3. 80% of all our consumption is based on habit – it should be based on need.

4. Junk food alters our flavor perception – that disrupts the choices we make.

5. Processed food alters our appetite – and fools our system into consuming what it shouldn't.

6. We are what we eat – you get that, right?

7. Food alters the body at the cellular level – fasting returns it to its original state.

8. It is better to look at things from a perspective of balance – than to look at it in absolute terms.

9. Not everyone can, nor should everyone, fast for extended periods, but everyone can fast for short periods.

10. Fasting is a mind game, no matter how much you feel the body revolt.

Just keep these ten things in mind and they will come in handy over the time you alter your life to embrace the practices of intermittent fasting.

Chapter 1: Our Relationship with Food

There are two ways that we can see food. We can see it is as a source of nutrition and energy, or we can see it as a source of pleasure. Seeing it as both are a great way to live, but, unfortunately, we have all fallen into the pit of putting pleasure first at the expense of its primary purpose. Doing it once, then again, and then the third time is enough to alter the habits of more than 66% of the adult population and more than 86% of the kids' population.

Think about that for a minute. It does not take much to alter your taste senses to form bad eating habits. Corporate giants like General Mills and P&G and the rest know it. They have the secret sauce. They know that if they add x amount of salt, y amount of fat and z amount of sugar, the person they are targeting gets hooked on it for life. That's the concoction – salt, sugar, and fat. The ratios are specific, but a highly guarded secret developed by the multi-million-dollar labs that are operated like a spy outfit. The reason is that that formula translates to billions in revenues for everything from potato chips to frozen pizza. Almost everything we eat, whether it's from fast-food outlets, sit-down restaurants, even many grocery items, have been engineered for taste and addiction to the point that it blunts our most crucial feature – to have the appetite for the things we need to eat – not the desire for the things that give us pleasure.

To understand how it works, and how it affects us, and why intermittent fasting is the best program to reverse all this; we need to start with the basics of how our body uses and replenishes energy and nutrients.

We Are What We Eat – Literally

We are driven by a sophisticated genetic algorithm that determines a hub of physiological patterns in us. Each of us has an almost unique pattern of this physiology and that affects the kinds of foods we are attracted to. When you add culture, geography, and climate to the mix, it alters the equation even more.

An experiment was conducted in Scandinavia where an already-deceased animal was irradiated and buried beside a group of trees. Another group of plants was kept in pots at the same average distance from the burial site. A year later, they took samples from various parts of the trees and from the plants that were in the pots. The potted plants were a control group to see how much of radiation would reach the trees, even though they were not physically sharing the same soil. There were extremely low levels – almost imperceptible levels in the potted plants. In the trees that shared the soil with the buried radioactive carcass, detectable levels of radiation could be found in all parts of the trees, all the way to the canopy of the tree.

I will get to the reason for this anecdote in a minute.

In research conducted in a small village 250 miles north of Tokyo, near the port of Kesennuma, they found that there was an abnormally high rate of mercury occurrence in the village's population. It turns out that Kesennuma, which is the largest fishing port specializing in shark-fin, was selling shark meat cheaply because the real prize in the shark is the fin that is exported as a delicacy to neighbors like China and Taiwan. This village with high mercury incidence was consuming a lot of the fish because it was the cheapest thing in the market and ingesting high levels of mercury.

The point of the last two anecdotes is to convince you, if you aren't already, that we are what we eat in more ways than most people realize. What you eat, drink and inhale enter your body and then make their way deep within you, some even lodging itself at a cellular level.

The good news is that, given time, what we ingest will also egress. For instance, if I drink a cup of water, that cup of water eventually makes its way out of me. If I drink a cup of tea, the solutes in the water that enters my body makes its way through my bloodstream, some of it may enter some of my cells, or go through some kind of reaction and then it eventually exits my body as well. It is the process of metabolism, the process of extracting energy while breaking down sources of energy. The body extracts energy, and it extracts nutrients from everything that we consume.

Did you know that we could actually eat cardboard, and it will provide us with some energy? The conversion won't be efficient, and the energy required to break it down would be excessive, but it won't be zero either, but energy is not the only thing that we need. We need nutrients as well. Nutrients are just elements, molecules, and compounds that are used in the rebuilding and replenishing of tired and old cells.

Even ingesting a toxin (if below a certain threshold) will make us ill (even violently so) but then, in time, our body returns to normal. Think about getting intoxicated after a wild night of drinking. The hangover kicks in the following morning, but eventually, the body works to return itself to a normal state. In the same way, eating junk food occasionally is not good for you, but your body will find a way to correct itself if you stop long enough because what you eat starts to break down and is expunged. Even some of the damage that it may have caused is repaired as the body seeks to return to its baseline.

Regenerative by Design

The one fact that you must remember about our body is that it is in a constant state of generation and a constant state of degeneration. As a young child, our generative pace is significantly more than our degenerative, and that causes growth. It's like filling a water bucket that has a hole. If you fill it with more water than is exiting it, the water level increases.

As time progresses, that balance shifts in the body. It starts off being more generative than degenerative, to being equally balanced throughout most of adulthood. That's the time we stop growing, but the regeneration continues and so does the degeneration. What happens is that what is used and old is expelled and the new replaces it. The oldest cell in your body at any point in time is no more than two years of age; most of the time they are less than six weeks old.

Then you come to the time when degeneration exceeds regeneration and this is when there is increased cell death and reduced function and less repair, and so the end effect is shrinkage and reduced operational efficacy. It's like the leak in the bucket is letting out more water than the faucet is filling it up with. Eventually, regeneration totally ceases and the degenerative process continues until… well, you get the picture.

Regeneration requires a couple of things to come together. The first is that you have to provide your body with the elements it needs to regenerate. Take, for instance, the iron in your blood. Iron is a critical element in your system. Its task is to bind with oxygen molecules and transport them to areas in the body that have a low concentration of oxygen. If you deplete your iron but don't replace it, you will slowly become less efficient at carrying oxygen, and that could lead to tiredness, lethargy, confusion and so on. To remedy the situation, you have to consume iron, and you have to consume the kinds that are better absorbed by the body, and the iron that is better absorbed is called the heme irons, which typically come from animal sources.

Iron is naturally depleted and is replaced by the iron we consume. Now, imagine if we stop consuming these sources of iron, what happens in time? Slowly, we begin to have insufficient iron levels to supply us with the oxygen we need to operate at the level we have to on a daily basis. That eventually leads to other complications.

As part of a balanced nutritional intake, we need to absorb iron from the things we eat. But, let's say we fill up on things that have no nutrition, in this case, iron. What happens?

To answer that, you need to know this: When you have an iron deficiency (just for this example) it creates an appetite of the foods that have heme iron in it. Your body knows how to trigger the appetite for the food it needs, and if you follow along and give in to your appetite (only in this case), your body gets exactly what it is looking for and all is well. But, if you neglect it, and only interpret the appetite as hunger, then you may neglect the request for iron-containing food and instead eat something that has a low-iron content or no iron at all. In this case, even if you are eating a nutritious meal, it's still junk food because you are taking in calories above what you need, but not the nutrient your body is looking for.

Here comes a problem. What if, with your sense of appetite so confused, it doesn't 'hear' the call for that steak or baked clams (both of which contain iron)? What happens is that you just go on and eat what you've been programmed to eat and you get your calories and nutrition that is maybe stored, but, for the most part, you don't get what the body needs on that particular day, and so you find yourself 'hungry' a little while later.

This is a problem because you've already taken in a dose of calories to satisfy your caloric needs, but, since you haven't satisfied your nutritional needs, your body is going to want more food, food that contains the nutrient it needs. Since you can't tell what that is, you take a stab at eating some more and you gain more calories but not the nutrient needed. You can obviously see where the needle on this scale is going.

That's the general consensus of eating habits in this country. We eat so much junk that our bodies never get the nutrition it needs and so we stay hungry, only to consume more empty calories.

If you're wondering how the body knows to ask for steak or clams (or whatever it is your source of iron is), here is the answer: Since birth, the mind is recording all the ingredients it consumes and what floor it was attached to. Your body associates flavor with nutrients and, when you have a deficiency, the body gives you the appetite for that particular flavor. If you fuel the appetite correctly, then you are rewarded with a balanced meal. If you are not, then you will end up taking on empty calories. What has all this to do with intermittent fasting? Everything.

The first thread we need to pull on here is appetite and palette. Remember that your body will bring the deficiency to your attention. If you pay heed, then all is well, but, if you can't hear or recognize this whisper, you're not going to be able to do anything about it. Intermittent fasting returns the body to a state where you can accurately recognize what the body needs at any particular point in time. You stop craving the junk food, if you chose to do so, and you start getting in touch with your own state of health.

This is the main reason you see many of the websites and e-books telling you how people on the program start to lose their wrinkles, because the body gets the nutrients it needs to keep the skin as elastic as possible; it rejuvenates. This is the reason people report that the diet rids them of blurry vision because the body gets the nutrients it needs to fix most forms of ocular degeneration, and the list goes on.

Let's get back to the underlying mechanisms of the body and the relationship it grows to create with food.

The body, and, by extension, your appetite is a function of a nicely tuned balance. Food, with their natural flavors, gives you clues as to what is in them and your subconscious picks up on that.

Junk Food

Why do we eat so much junk? Because the trifecta of flavor - salt, sugar and fat, kidnaps our senses and holds us hostage, but if we use this definition, then virtually all the food we eat can be considered junk. It's not just snacks that are engineered, even convenient TV dinners and ready-made meals are engineered for taste instead of nutrition, and rightfully so because they are a business and their job, by definition, is to give you what you will keep coming back for. It's not their fault, it's the consumer's.

But wait, it's not really your fault as a consumer either. Even if the consumer made the conscious decision to eat healthily, it would be almost impossible to do so without going through significant difficulty. Imagine not being able to eat out, or not being able to enjoy the tastes that you have grown accustomed to. Being alive is partially about enjoying life, and totally cutting out these pleasures is not the answer. You want to be able to eat your cake and have it too. You want to enjoy your meal and remain healthy at the same time.

Most people live on either extreme. They either completely change their lifestyle, becoming vegetarians, vegans, or perpetually condition themselves to live on a cornucopia of fad diets. I used to do that. I lived on the no-carb diet once. It was great at first, my chubby handles peeled right off in three weeks, and I was energized and had clarity of thought, but then, after a few weeks, the maintenance diet got old. My psyche was arcing back to the norm. What about discipline, you ask? Well, I had tons of that, and I kept in line but I was not happy. There was no more to gain, yet the maintenance diet had me sacrificing so much for nothing in return.

Then I tried the Paleo diet, and that worked really great too, but, after a while, it was a lifestyle change and the heart does indeed grow fonder of the things that you deprive it of, especially the ones that don't make the consequences apparent right away.

Like the first two, I tried many of the diets that were available and I have to say that they all worked. There really wasn't anything wrong with them, except there was prolonged sacrifice from things that I enjoyed.

Then I came across fasting. Not just intermittent fasting, but fasting in general. Fasting changes you in ways that you can only understand when you experience it. Fasting changes you from the inside out and then renews your mind, body, and spirit.

The best part is that it works for everyone. Fasting allows the body to rest. Think of it this way. If you take a moment and look at your relationship with food as an intimate one, where eating is there to sustain you, to give you pleasure and to act as a medium to share with loved ones, a holistic look at food, then you must realize that balance is key rather than completely swearing off certain foods, even if your body is craving something it needs.

We eat too much, not just because of the pleasure of taste. We eat too much because of our habit of eating three meals (plus snacks) when we don't need all that food. Breakfast lunch and dinner are scheduled to make nutrition intake regular and timely, but we don't need all that. A woman's body only needs 2,000 calories per day. In a week, that's only 14,000 calories. If we can stuff our entire nutritional intake into that caloric count, then we have no issues of overeating.

Holistic Perspective

Well, ok you can't really say 'holistic' and then make it a perspective because holistic means all perspectives combined into one comprehensive understanding but, for now, let's just go with the term because it conveys the notion that you can't just look at the relationship between food and humans from one perspective. Think about art for a second, as a metaphor for your total self – the paper, the pan, the frame, the sketch, the artist, even the humidity of the air that surrounds it, or the medium of the paint be it oil or gouache. When one gazes at the painting, they see an image and that's all but, when you experience a painting holistically, you start to understand all the elements that came together at that one moment in time and froze into a manifestation of the artist's inspiration.

That same relationship applies to you and food. The way you look and feel, your aggregate health, your levels of motivation, and your potential are all a function of the things that become a part of you; the food that you put in you, just like all the things that go into a painting. That holistic perspective of food is one that is necessary so that you can give it the food it needs when it needs it. Memorizing food pyramids and looking at diet books all pale in comparison to heeding the clarion call sounded by your own body but, to heed the call, you have to hear it first. For you to hear it, you need your senses in top notch and that allows you to hear, then heed the call your body makes.

Most people get numbed and lulled by habits that prevent them from hearing the call. The shouting of the reinforced habits to consume salt, sugar and fat far exceed the whisper of the body's needs. Our taste buds ride roughshod over our nutritional needs and we end up on the path to obesity and ill-health.

As such, is the solution to get highly disciplined with food? Well, you can do it that way, but absolutism in dietary conditions is not the best answer. You are, after all, living to enjoy all that this life has to offer. Eat up, drink up, smoke it too if you have to, but the thing is that you can't do more of one thing than your body is able to handle.

Let me give you an example. I smoked two packs a day for fifteen years, and then I quit only because I didn't feel like it anymore. Three years later, I was at the doctor's for a scheduled scan and the doctor didn't know that I had smoked. My lungs were clean. Two reasons that happened – one: the body cleans up whatever trash you put into it – if you give it enough time. Two: fasting expedites the clean-up process.

Intermittent fasting does two beneficial things for you, and we will look at all this in greater detail as the rest of the book unfolds: first, it gives your body the chance to catch up and process the junk that you take in in the name of taste and pleasure; second, it gives your senses the time to reset your palate.

The objective of this books is to leave you with a path to effective intermittent fasting. You can think of it as the base of the pyramid which supports the rest of your existence and culinary experience.

First, the strategy and healthy approach to intermittent fasting will give you the tools you need to prepare your mind and body to purge all that is disrupting your health.

Second, we will look at the implementation of intermittent fasting. Many people can jump straight into it and not feel the effects, but most people will not be able to reap the benefits of the program if they do not implement it correctly.

Finally, we will look at the way to maintain intermittent fasting and/or combine it with other fasting programs to be able to experience added benefits.

With these three steps and the tools of discipline and purpose, there is no reason to not be able to shift your body into perfect shape and tune your state into one that is vibrant and powerful.

Chapter 2: Six Physiological Effects of Intermittent Fasting

In the book, we talk about a number of different effects that you will experience from the changes in taste and control over your habits. This chapter overlaps that but looks exclusively at the physiological aspects of intermittent fasting. It is based on personal experience and scientific research that has been conducted in numerous universities. To form a proper foundation, we need to look at some of the body's systems and the chemistry that is involved. Don't worry; it will not get too involved.

Insulin

Insulin is the primary anabolic peptide hormone that is produced in the pancreatic islets by beta cells. The primary purpose of insulin is to attach itself to sugar and then unlock cells in the body to allow the entry of the sugar. Without insulin, cells would not be able to accept sugar and thus they would not be able to function. In Type 1 Diabetes, the pancreatic islets do not produce insulin and so patients need to inject themselves. In Type 2, the body develops a resistance to insulin and the effect is the same. There is one other effect of insulin that you should add to this. When insulin is released, it promotes the storage of energy in adipose tissue, and it suppresses the use of adipose tissue in energy conversion. There are two parts of this that you need to understand. The first is that the more sugar you ingest, the more insulin you are going to release, which will then lead to two scenarios. The first is that you may become resistant to it and have to take injections. The second is that even if you are resistant, it doesn't mean that there are no insulin hormones in your bloodstream; there is, but you are not able to metabolize the sugar. What additionally happens is that the insulin blocks energy conversion from fat cells.

Fasting drops your sugar levels (assuming you do not load up when you get back to eating). When your sugar levels drop, inulin secretion is reduced. Two things happen here; the first is that you do not become resistant to insulin, and second, there is nothing preventing your fat cells from being converted to energy. If your fat is blocked from converting to energy, then they will always remain and there is no other way you can lose weight.

Intermittent fasting is not designed to be a one-off and lose some weight here and there. It is designed to modify your physiological processes and change the way your body does things. In this case, it is designed to alter your insulin profile and your energy derivation profile (where you get your energy from).

It is a well-documented fact that insulin resistance (Type II Diabetes) can be avoided or even reversed in some cases after extended intermittent fasting.

Human Growth Hormone (Somatotropin)

The human growth hormone, HGH, is triggered during periods of fasting. This is an evolutionary aspect of the human body. When we are hungry or starving, our body needs to get itself in gear to hunt and satisfy that hunger. The natural state of the human body is to hunt and devour. Contrary to some belief, it is not designed to sit back and be served. The more you hustle and move, the more your body becomes fine-tuned. When HGH is released, it does two things: first, it helps to expedite the repair of tissue; and second, it helps to regenerate old tissue. HGH also expedites the metabolism of muscular fat. When you fast intermittently, your body gets into the habit of releasing HGH and that allows you to repair your cells, keeping yourself more adept at burning energy. It also promotes the use of fat in energy creation. In essence, the HGH keeps you feeling young and healthy. It also does quite a bit for the elasticity of your skin, and the strength of your bones. HGH has a simple profile. It is found in higher quantities when you are young to promote growth in height and weight. As you get older, it starts to decrease and then it is only sufficient to help with the repair and replacement of degrading cells. Taking supplement HGH is not always the best solution, but stimulating the HGH within your body helps at a cellular level and, more importantly, it helps with the metabolism of fat.

Increased Metabolic Rate

Without getting into the biochemistry of metabolism, it will be suffice to say that when you stretch out your eating schedule, as when you do when you practice intermediate fasting, your body increases its metabolic rate. The body is designed to operate effectively and efficiently when it runs on a lean diet. When it eats too much, the body needs to spend a lot of its time digesting food and shuttling it to various areas and, when in excess, has to convert it to fat and store it. This directs much of the resources away from what you could otherwise be doing. Have you ever finished Thanksgiving dinner and felt drowsy? Happens to me every year, and I let it as it is one of those times that feeling that brand of bliss is ok in my book. A cocktail of hormones: melatonin, tryptophan, and serotonin are released after meals and this gets you in that drowsy state. The purpose behind that is to put you in a state of rest while your body digests and puts the calories and nutrients away. On average, during intermittent fasting, your body will increase its metabolism by 10%.

Mental Acuity and Strength

To keep you in a state of rest, the shot of hormones places your mind in a relaxed state and that reduces your mental acuity. It's primal in its design. Cavemen that needed to go out and hunt were given the extra boost in mental acuity and strength when they were hungry but turned sleepy and relaxed after a full meal. We, today, are no different. It has been researched and observed that intermittent fasting accelerates and prolongs the neural development in the brain.

Intermittent fasting stimulates the release of Brain-Derived Neurotrophic factor (BDNF). This is a hormone instrumental in motivating the body and staving off any form of depression. When expressed periodically, it can boost your abilities. When expressed continuously, it will change your life.

Reduced Oxidation and Aging Stress

It is now well documented that the oxidation leads to things like heart disease and stroke by leading to the hardening of arteries and blood vessels. Oxidative stress also alters gene expression and the regulation of tissue repair. That has a direct impact on how your cells age as you want them to be flexible and elastic. That results in better looking skin and, when you do lose weight your skin will not sag because it is properly nourished.

Reduced Risk of Heart Disease

Intermittent fasting improves LDL levels, which has a direct impact on cardiovascular health. That, in turn, has an impact on blood pressure which is directly responsible for kidney health. This is done in two ways. First of all, it reduces the stress in your heart to keep working at digesting large quantities of food and storing energy in the fat cells. If you use what you take in, there is no need to put your heart through that stress. Ask anyone who is out of shape and on the larger side of life, how they feel after a meal – they will tell you they need to rest. Many need a cup of coffee. The coffee is to get caffeine into your system and push blood to your brain so that you get the energy you need. A better way would be to not eat so much. Don't look to be full and don't look to be satiated.

The second way your heart is helped is by the reduced oxidation rates in your blood vessels like you read in the previous paragraph. When your heart has to work harder while you work out, then your heart is also getting the proper workout.

Chapter 3: Preparing for the Intermittent Fast

There are three steps you need to take before you get started on your fast. It is preparatory in nature and is not considered as part of the actual fast, but is highly important, nonetheless. Consider it as the warm-up phase. Just as any athletic activity requires a period of stretching and priming before an exercise, fasting too requires that you prime your body. Let's break this down into two parts. We will first talk about the physical priming and then we will follow this with the psychological priming.

Physical Priming

Physical priming is accomplished over a series of tasks that will ready your body for the fast. It is different from the psychological priming in that this covers the physical acts that you have to perform, or refrain from, in order to prepare the biological and physiological process of the body. Many of the body's systems are based on habit and anticipation. To make sweeping changes without altering the habit and anticipation profile of your present condition would be cause for much grief, discomfort, and pain. That will eventually lead to the cessation of the diet, fast or new regiment. Worst of all, that will result in a negative impression to the objective and a resistance to try it again. After all, if something doesn't work, why would we want to try it again?

As such, to avoid that, you should be willing to patiently put off the actual start of the fasting process and spend a good amount of time preparing yourself.

Step One

This step assumes that you are considering intermittent fasting from a holistic perspective; to improve mind, body, and spirit, in addition to trimming a few pounds off your frame. Being holistic in your approach has a compounding effect. Better consumption results in better energy levels, leading to better activity levels, which, in turn, release brain altering hormones that invigorate and motivate, and that causes better activity levels. Once you get going, it changes your life, if you allow it to.

The removal of toxins in your body is a given in any and all weight loss and fasting programs. When you burn fat, toxins that are stored within the adipose tissue structure are released into the body. That has an effect, but it needs to be flushed out, and if you continue with the intermittent fasting, you will find that there are some days in the induction period that you feel down and out. It is to be expected. You just have to grab the rails and hold on.

I've mentioned in my other hardcore fasting books about a specific case that illustrates this. A reformed hallucinogen addict had gained a tremendous amount of weight over the course of his addiction due to unrelated medical issues. When common medicine failed to assist with a problem he was having, he turned to an ancient Ayurveda medicine and herbalism. To prepare him for the regimen, the doctor put him on a water-lemon diet for seven days. During this time, his only sustenance was seven parts water and one part diluted lemon juice. In other words, he was supposed to keep an eye on the amount of water he ingested. He could have as much as he wished, whenever he felt like it. The only practice he had to adhere to was that either glass would have to be the juice of half a lemon diluted with water to taste and consume, and then he would go back to drinking water again after that. The lemon juice kept his electrolyte balance in check.

At the end of the fourth day and into the fifth, with visible signs of weight loss, he also began to hallucinate. According to him, it felt almost like the effect of the hallucinogens he used to ingest, but with a slightly less intensity. That lasted for four days. When he came out from it, he was feeling alert, fresh, and significantly lighter.

The hallucinogens, just like other toxins, get stored in pockets within your fat layer under the skin. As the fat is metabolized and reintroduced into the system, these pockets are punctured and re-enter your bloodstream causing the same effects as they were originally designed to do. Be prepared for that as you undertake your fast.

The reason this fact is introduced into the conversation today is that the step that you have to accomplish in the beginning has to do with the cessation of certain habits when it comes to food and activity. It's not like you have to give up coffee or something like that, but there are some foods you should give up and certain activities you should perform which will allow you to reap the best benefits of intermittent fasting.

Yes, there are many advocates of IF that will tell you that there is nothing to give up and that the IF is more about a lifestyle than a diet. This is true; however, altering your diet profile to a limited extent will prove to be extremely beneficial. The preparation phase requires you to remove your body from the routine that it has at the molecular level. Think about it this way. If you consume high quantities of salt, then three things happen: First, you develop a tolerance for it in taste so that, over time, you will need more salt in your food to give it the taste that is pleasing; and, second, your hydration level will change and this will make your cells operate at reduced efficiency. Finally, your electrolytes will alter in concentration because the salt will displace some of the electrolytes.

The point of this is to show you that each action has a cascade of consequences. Just altering your regular intake of salt can change your body and knock it off its equilibrium. Even when you realize that salt is not good for you and you stop or reduce the intake, your initial reaction is not necessarily of health but you could feel unwell until your body reaches its new equilibrium.

The body is about balance and so one needs to remember that all changes will alter that balance. It's like the cessation of smoking. Even though smoking is bad for you, when you quit, it feels horrible for months. That's because your body is thrown off equilibrium and is struggling to return to it.

These are just the illustration of the concept of balance and equilibrium. In intermittent fasting, the changes you are about to make will alter your equilibrium and you have to prepare for that. Step one is about reducing the things that will aid in the reaching of that balance.

In step one, you need to reduce three key elements from your system so that your body gets on the path faster. The first element is processed sugar. I am not here to judge you on your sugar intake. It is best if you keep your sugar intake as natural as possible, especially to one that has a low glycemic index. Second, reduce table salt to zero and substitute it with sea salt. Not all salts are created equal. Table salt is chemically made and alters your body chemistry adversely. Sea salt, on the other hand, is natural and balances the electrolytes in your body rather than displacing it. Third, eliminate synthetic oils from your diet, especially ones that are hydrogenated.

So, what has eliminating three foods from your intake have to do with the intermittent fast?

Everything!

The fast itself is not about reducing foods, or classes of foods, but is about altering your consumption schedule. The reason behind reducing the three groups above is to make the times that you are off food to become easier to manage. It will also make you a healthier person.

In many cases, unhealthy foods prompt the craving to eat. Have you ever been on a junk food binge or diet? After a while, that's all you want to eat because of the perfectly engineered salt-sugar-fat trifecta. It will take about two weeks to get your body rebalanced. During the execution of this step, there is no other element of the fact that you need to practice. Eat just as you always have. When starting a new fast or diet program, it is important to change one thing at a time and not change all aspects concurrently.

Step Two

Water.

We could leave it at that since it makes all the sense in the world, but a little more illumination on this matter is necessary. On average, the human adult's body consists of 60% water by weight so, if you weigh 160 lbs, 96 lbs of that is water, but that's not really the point here. In this case, water is your composition, but the reason you need to consume large quantities of water, aside from not getting dehydrated, is to use it as a flush. It's just like flushing the radiator of your car. Water is the best thing there is to flush the human body at the cellular level.

Just note that you shouldn't drink highly purified (or Reverse Osmosis) water. This is not healthy. You should drink purified mineral water or you should add electrolytes to highly purified water. If the water has zero mineral content, it will leach minerals from your body.

Your preliminary stage, or preparing your body, is to hydrate it well and begin the body's journey into flushing out the toxins that will make any fast difficult. The initial period when you are in the process of ridding yourself of the salt, sugar, and fat, is the hardest psychologically. If you do not have a sufficient water intake, it wouldn't be an effective flushing process.

Adequate water will increase metabolism at the cellular level, carry the flushed toxins out at a faster rate, and improve the metabolism rates. Don't confuse this step with the consumption of water during the fast. Remember, at this stage, you are still on a normal diet. You have not begun the actual alteration of your intake schedule.

Step Three

Walk more. Before you start the intermittent fast, it is best that you start off by walking, if you do not already. If you already walk a lot, increase the inclination of your path, or increase the pace. If you do not already walk, start a daily routine of walking for at least thirty minutes daily. This will jump start your metabolism.

When you begin intermittent fasting, walking will magnify the change and the weight loss. Walking is a different ball game than its more strenuous cousins – running and swimming. Aerobic walking is a game changer and it will expedite and magnify the fruits of your IF.

The more you walk, the more you will promote aerobic metabolism and circulation. As your metabolism and circulation improve, your body will become more efficient at toxin elimination and you will be able to regulate your energy levels and your weight will start to melt away.

Psychological Priming

The second most important thing that you need to do before you get started with the intermittent fasting is to prepare yourself psychologically. If you are not serious about this, then your old habits will get the better of you. Everything you do is a matter of habit, from the toothpaste you prefer to the fact that you brush your teeth at a given point each morning. Your body is a manifestation of habits. Even your sugar and salt consumption is a habit.

Habits are as much psychological as they are chemical and physical. The chemical version is the rewards distributed by the neurotransmitters every time a habit is completed. You know that feeling of doing what you are used to doing, and the agony of missing something that you always do. When you start to fast intermittently, your body needs to break a habit that it has been used to for ages. That becomes a problem.

Most people know of Pavlov's Dog. It was an experiment conducted by physiologist Ivan Pavlov to prove conditioning and habit. In the experiment, he rang a bell each time he fed the dog and, after some time, he found that ringing the bell alone was sufficient to get the dog to anticipate the arrival of food.

By doing this, he showed that one can be conditioned into associative behavior. In the dog's case, he showed signs of appetite when the bell rang. In humans, we get hungry at a certain time of day because we are conditioned to eat breakfast, lunch and dinner and sometimes have an afternoon snack. The problem is that we live in a culture of unhealthy eating. We pay more attention to timing than we do need. We also pay more attention to pleasure than we do nutrition. These two put together, alter our affinity for healthy food and to a healthy diet.

To be able to take the IF to its furthest extent of benefit, we need to prime the way we look at food and the habits that we have formed. To this end, we have three steps that need to be considered.

Step One

Find a new activity to replace the old. Say, for instance, if you are going to start skipping lunch, then the best way to do that is to replace your lunch routine with something different. Some people replace their lunch hour with a session at the gym. If you have a gym close by, then that works great. If you have a friend that you can go with, that is even better. You will soon be able to get over your habit. That's an example, but, like that, the idea is to get your mind off the event of eating.

Be warned though, it will take some time for you to stop feeling hungry at that time because your conditioning has been to have lunch, and this is one of the oldest habits you have had. Since kindergarten, you have been conditioned to have a meal when the sun hits its zenith. Replacing your lunchtime slot, or whichever meal you plan on skipping with another activity, is one of the things that will keep you on the path to success with this fast.

Step Two

Rearrange your home so that the kitchen and living area are different. There is an old trick to quit smoking – go on vacation and quit while you are there. The reasoning behind it is that you will be able to trick your system into overcoming the habit because the triggers are partially gone. In the same way, if you alter the way your dining area and living area are, then it will change the way you slide down the path to a meal time. This works especially well if you are planning to skip dinners, although dinners at home are the hardest to do because it is usually when the entire family gets together for a meal and it is more than just food at that time. So dinners are hard to do.

Even if you chose to skip lunch, changing the way you move around your home alters the energy of your home in such a way you will feel anew.

Step Three

Now, this is going to sound like a strange one, but it works. Change your dressing. It is a great way to hack your brain. If your brain sees a different you, it feels different and then it will ease into the new routine.

That's the six steps you need to think about and perform. The physical priming is something that you will have to do before you start intermittent fasting, but the psychological priming, you can start before or during the intermittent fasting.

Chapter 4: Intermittent Fasting

Remember, intermittent fasting is not about hunger or starving yourself, it's about changing the frequency of your meals and making your food intake intermittent instead of frequent. This is predicated on the fact that your body does not need food all the time – that is conditioning. Your parents and teachers taught you that, and their parents and teachers before them taught them that, so it goes back generations. If you can get that conditioned habit out of the way, then you will realize that your body doesn't really need to take in lots of food. Even the way it stores and uses those stores changes when you stop feeding it every four hours.

Beginners' Fasting

Up to this point, you have prepared your body for this next step – the point where you begin your actual fasting. It is Day One – D1. There are three variations of D1 depending on which meal you plan on skipping. If you plan on skipping breakfast more often than other meals, then your IF plan is going to take a unique route to your goal. Not everyone can do this. If you don't tailor the IF plan according to your body, then some of you are going to come away from trying this and thinking this doesn't work. It does if you match it to your body type. Some of you are best suited to skipping breakfast, some of you aren't. If you have the ability to skip breakfast, then you will be able to switch your body's reliance on food as energy and get your body to burn fat in the liver and fat tissue for energy instead.

A quick recap before we get into the actual fasting - intermittent fasting does three things for you:

- First, it reduces the total number of calories that you accumulate. Men typically need about 2,200 calories if they live a sedentary lifestyle, while women need about 2,000 but, three square meals in a day ends up giving you a lot more than that if you aren't calorie counting. It takes 3,500 calories above what you need for your lifestyle to put on a one pound weight. Americans consume an average of 3,600 calories per day.

- What this means, in practical terms, is that if you consume 3,000 calories per day and you only need 2,000, this means you have 1,000 calories above your need that is converted to fat. In one week, you will have an excess of 7,000 calories and that means you would have gained two pounds.

- If you use the same maths and calculate that for the average American, what you have is 3,600 minus 2,000, which gives you 1,600 calories in excess of daily needs. In a week, that works out to be 11,200 calories in excess of requirements. Since every 3,500 calories work out to be a pound in weight, that makes the average weekly weight gain in America to be just a little over three pounds a week. This is beyond unhealthy. Carrying extra weight is one thing, but crowding out the essential nutrients because you are displacing it with junk, deprives your body of the elements it needs to repair itself. So, on one hand, you are asking your body to do more work and, on the other hand, you are depriving it of the elements it needs to replace and repair the body. It's a double whammy.

- Another thing is that it alters the reaction time it takes your body to switch between drawing energy from the food you just ate, to drawing energy from the glycogen in your muscle and liver. When your body has no more food in its gastrointestinal environment, it switches to the glycogen in your muscles and liver. Your muscles will give you about 1,500 calories worth of energy and your liver will give you an additional 400 calories. In total, you have about 2,000 calories worth of energy stored as glycogen. That essentially means that you can go an entire day without eating and still have the calories you need to get through the day because your body will switch its source of fuel from the sugars in your stomach to the glycogen in your muscles and liver. The switching process is uncomfortable if you are not used to it and IF will train your body to get used to it and switch faster.

- Next! IF allows you to eat what you want by controlling when you eat. As long as it is not unhealthy, you don't really need to cut your meals down and feel unsatisfied. After all, part of eating is the enjoyment of it. You don't really need to count your calories. What you do need to do is cut out the engineered food and eat what is naturally appealing to you.

The point of intermittent fasting is to get you to peak health and, to do that, it is designed to alter the way you see food and the way your body treats it. That, in turn, returns you to your ideal weight and boosts your energy profile to an optimal level. In order to get to this point, you need to trigger the body's ability to switch to burning glycogen then burning fat.

Chapter 5: Induction Week Practice and Meal Plan

You begin with an empty day, and we call this your pre-intermittent fast. On this day, you are focused on the cleansing process. It is meant to gradually rid your system of toxins and the overpowering nature of sugar, fats, and salt. The best way to do this is to completely wipe out food for the better part of the day.

Pre-Intermittent Fast

This is when you wipe out all food from sunrise to sunset. Wake up in the morning and have a glass of water that has been sitting on your side table since the night before. The water should be at a temperature that is not warmer or colder than you can handle; room temperature will not shock your system.

Go for your walk. If you have to get to work, then get up a half hour earlier and get out for the brisk walk. If you are in the habit of going to the gym, then start your routine with a half hour walk on the treadmill. Do not run, walk fast or brisk. Inhale with your nose and exhale with your mouth. Drink as much water as you want during the workout and, at the end of the workout, have lemon mixed with that water and drink that. You have to rebalance your electrolytes.

You need to make sure that you consume between 2 and 3 liters of water every day depending on your lifestyle. Make sure you have a proper intake of electrolytes as well (that's the purpose of the lemon), and then get to work and find something to do during lunch. Don't end up sitting at your desk or tagging along with your friends who go out for lunch. Either get back to the gym or go to the park. Do not put yourself near food. When you get home, have more water and go to sleep. If you have been drinking enough, you should feel a little tired and you will be missing your meals, but don't give in to your mind.

Rationalizing

Your first day is about breaking the habit of food schedules and making you hungry. Yes, you should get hungry and feel hunger for what it is. It's not designed to make you miserable or make you ill. If you are hyper or hypoglycemic, then check with your doctor before doing this. It is also designed so that your senses return to the baseline and a sudden change to the intake schedule helps with that.

By the next morning, you would have been without food for almost 36 hours. Don't tell your mind that, as it's not going to allow you to do it. Just get up, make a decision, and then do it. Distract your mind for as long as you can. At this point, you have burned over 2,300 calories, including your additional walk and the number of calories you burn in your sleep. With zero caloric intake, those calories came from your glycogen stores in your liver and muscles. Those stores amount to approximately 2,000 calories. If you've burned

2,300 in the last 36 hours without any intake, you have gone through those glycogen stores and started to convert fat to energy. When you wake up the following morning, the hardest part of the fast would have past because you were asleep.

While you sleep, your body will burn 0.4 calories per hour per pound. This is for all your body's functions. For instance, you weigh 150 pounds and sleep for 7 hours, that would mean that you would burn 0.4 calories x 7 hours x 150 lbs = 420 calories.

That extra 420 calories would have triggered your body to change metabolic pathways and begin the process of getting energy from fat.

Now you are ready to get to breakfast.

Day One

As soon as you wake up, you will realize that you are still alive and you are not in as bad a shape as you thought you might be. Everything is fine, and you have just technically been without food for 36 hours just because you fasted from dawn to dusk.

Start with yogurt. If you like steak, you are welcome to it. If you fancy fruit, go for it. You can have whatever you feel like having as long as it is not processed. The food you have cannot have sugar or sweetener. You can have lots of fruit, but it has to be ones that have a low glycemic index, preferably ones that have a GI less than 45. These can be cherries, dry apricots, grapefruits, pears, and apples. All these have a glycemic index below 45.

You can eat all the vegetables you want, meat and dairy also have no restrictions, and you can even have fresh milk, preferably goat's milk. Remember, the only limitation is that you shouldn't have processed food to avoid taking sugar, salt and fat.

The one thing to note is that your stomach has been empty and when you put food in it, it shouldn't be too much at all. Any desire to overeat is coming from the brain, not the body's physiology and you should refrain from giving in to it for now.

The yogurt helps to rebalance the bacteria population in the gut, and that will increase nutrient absorption. Remember the lower calories you take in for the same amount of nutrients, the healthier you will be. Yogurt helps in this effort by increasing nutrient absorption.

Next comes lunch. Again, no processed foods. More yogurt for dessert would be good too. Yogurt ice-cream is fine as well. You can go for salads, fish, nuts, cheese, meat, chicken, beans and whatever you want. You can salt it lightly with sea salt, but not table salt. You can sweeten your drinks with Coconut Palm Sugar, which is a low glycemic index sugar (it has a GI score of 35).

During the induction week, your results would be better if you took food that had a higher nutrient to calorie ratio. Take, for instance, table sugar. It has almost 400 calories in 100 grams, but has absolutely no nutrients. On the other hand, if you took honey, you would get the sweetness that it imparts and the added benefit of Vitamin B6, niacin, thiamine, pantothenic acid, riboflavin, magnesium, sulfur, phosphorus, iron, calcium, chlorine, potassium, iodine, sodium, copper, and manganese. Honey is sweet, but it is not filled with empty calories. It is a good sweetener to have on hand.

One of the best things you can have for breakfast is steel cut oats. With only 200 calories in a serving, it brings the boost of polyphenols, selenium, phosphorus, manganese, and zinc.

Day Two

This is day 2 of your induction week to your intermittent fast. The most intense portion of this regimen is now behind you. You only had breakfast and lunch yesterday, and, as you wake up now, you have not had food for almost 20 hours.

Whatever difficulty you are feeling is being conjured by the mind because the mind has not fulfilled its sacred duty of performing its habits. As far as your body is concerned, it's doing great. This is a good time as any to come to terms with how involved your mind is with the way you eat and what you eat. When you go for your brisk walk, it's a good time to think about that.

The best way to knock back whatever the brain is feeling in terms of hunger is to get into a vigorous workout. If you are into aerobics or dancing, get moving this morning after your walk and you will find that the sweat and dopamine release is going to bat those feelings out of the park.

Drink lots of water because after breakfast today, you won't be having a meal until supper.

When you get to dinner, you would have been fasting for almost 12 hours. Your body is also burning more while it is awake and it has started to dip into your glycogen stores and perhaps even started to burn some fat.

But all that aside, with the end of the third day coming into view, the worst is now behind you. In most cases, you are going to wake up tomorrow and feel like a million bucks. You will even see some changes in your skin and your eyes should be clearer at this point.

Dinner on the third day should be anything you want as long as you remember to accomplish two things. The first is that you still shouldn't eat anything processed. That includes no fast food, boxed dinners or MSG. The second is that you don't overeat. You should never give yourself license to eat extra during a meal just because you skipped the last meal. Just so you are prepared, here is a snack recipe for days where you are more hungry than normal.

Snack Recipe

2 cups of oats

1 ½ ounces of raw sunflower seeds

3 ounces of crushed almonds

½ a cup of wheat germ

Vanilla extract, 2-3 drops

10 ounces of dried fruits of your choice - apricots, raisins, dried cranberries, cherries, or blueberries (you can use all of one variety or mix them up).

Get a non-stick pan and heat it until it is warm to the touch. Add five teaspoons of butter, and sauté the sunflower seeds and almonds in them, then add the oats.

This will soak up the butter. Mix in the dry fruits and the vanilla extract. Stir until all of them stick together, and then lay out on tin foil. Cover it, and then roll it. Press it down firmly so that you get a dense roll. Place that in the fridge. You can snack on this between any meals (but not during the fast period).

Just keep in mind that you are in the induction week and this is not how it will be once next week comes around. Your regular lifestyle won't be so intricate. It will be significantly easier. The snack recipe above will be a good source of fiber for you and it is something that you should always have as a snack, even in the weeks ahead. They will give you a good slow energy release and keep your insulin levels stable that way, and your fat tissue will not be precluded from being converted to energy.

Day Three

Your third day on the induction week should be one that is less stressful and more energized. You should start to feel a better flow of energy around you. You should observe the nature of that energy is now more constant through the day, and not periodically spiking right after meals and crashing a little while later. The oscillating nature of energy in fixed-meal time diets is no longer present and you will feel stable and that should be a source of peace. It is the day that you can go out for that walk and actually turn the return leg of it into a run. When you get back, you will have breakfast. Today, you will have breakfast and lunch and then you will fast until the following morning.

Have lunch by noon or 1pm at the latest, and then stop all food until the following day.

Day Four

This is the easiest day you will have until now. At this point, you will wake up and go for a walk. No need to top it off with a run, but you can take a long brisk walk if you feel like it. Your body will be coming to the realization that you do not need food every few hours to stay alive. Your mind also realizes that it likes the ketone-based energy it is getting for itself from the burning of ketone bodies during fat metabolization. You will be skipping breakfast, and, at this point, you won't even feel it. Get to lunch an hour later than you finished on day three. This means you have fasted for 24 hours straight. You should still be drinking no less than 2-3 liters of water in a day, and do not forget to add slices of lemon in the water to add to the electrolytes that you need to keep replenished.

If you have the sensation of a dry mouth at this point, don't be alarmed. It's not because you are drinking less than you should (if you have been drinking as mentioned). This is normal. Even if you get a coating on your tongue, just scrape it off. It is just the normal body process of clearing toxins from your body. As long as you are drinking at least 2 liters and you are urinating often, you are in good shape. Do not have dinner, but you can have a snack (the dry fruit bar we talked about earlier) three hours before you go to sleep.

Day Five

One of the things that you will start to notice is that you will sleep less. Your body has so much energy at this point that you will be more active and end up staying up longer. Try to keep your sleeping routine and wake up a little earlier if you find that your bed time is too early. That way you have a long day in the morning, but you can still get to bed early at night.

You should start bringing sea salt and honey, or coconut palm sugar into your recipes for flavor. Sea salt is a significantly better alternative than table salt, and it provides the electrolytes you need. Table salt doesn't. Coconut Palm Sugar is a better alternative to table sugar because it has a much lower Glycemic Index and will help you keep your insulin levels in check. Remember, insulin keeps fat cells from metabolizing.

Do your regular walk and workout to keep a normal day. You will be having lunch today. You can eat anything you feel like. Focus on what you feel like having. Stay away from thinking that everything looks or smells good. Stay home and look inside your fridge. What looks good to you? Do you feel like something colorful, something crunchy, or something creamy? All these sensations can give you a clue to what your body is asking for. Give your body what it wants. You will find that even the smallest portions of what the body needs will result in a feeling of being full.

It only takes a few days of disciplined conviction for your body to spring out of its faulty wiring. Within a week you will start to taste your food differently. You will find that eating is about what your body needs first, and then about pleasure second. You can still have food that brings pleasure, but do it in small portions and don't overdo it, and you will find that this week will pass in a flash.

Congratulations, it is now day six.

Day Six

You have only two days left and you will now get into the routine of real intermittent fasting. When you get on your regular day, intermittent fasting is about eating in windows and staying off of food at other times. You don't need to count calories, just listen to your body when it feels full. If you listen to your appetite, like when it feels like a burger or fish, or when it just wants a green salad, then you are giving your body all the food it needs and the nutrients that it is looking for. Once you are at that stage, you will find that you do not need to eat constantly. By this point, your body should have broken most of its habit of eating at prescribed times. That really is the whole point of this. There are three things that are the real points here:

1. Be independent of prescribed eating times.
2. Eat what your body tells you to eat.
3. Find pleasure and enjoyment in things other than food.

On the sixth day, what you will do is try one of two ways of doing the intermittent fast. Today, you will eat small portions of greens and fresh or dry fruits in single servings a few times during the day. Then have one large meal three hours before bed. That's your plan for the sixth day.

This is a good opportunity to bring fruits and vegetables into your diet and do it easily in digestible quantities. The first seven days also gets your body into the mode of burning stored fat so that you will enter the intermittent fasting period with a body that is in gear to burn fat.

Day Seven

You made it. You got to the last day of the induction period and you are ready to try one more fasting pattern. This one is simple. It's about giving yourself a four-hour window. In that window, you can eat whatever you want. The problem with it for some people is that they tend to binge eat. Don't do that. In a four-hour period, you should eat slowly. Start with something light. Yogurt is always good to have on a daily basis as it keeps your gut in optimal condition, followed by fruits and nuts, then followed by your main meal. Again, there are no restrictions except processed food.

The eating window can be at any time of the day. It can be from the time you wake up to four hours later, or it can be at mid-day. It can also be in a four-hour span, three hours before you get to bed. So, let's say you sleep at 10pm; three hours before that is 7pm. You should never eat just before getting to bed. Then, your eating window would be from 3pm to 7 pm. At the end of today, you have to make a choice. Figure out which of the two strategies you are going to try over the next week. You can always change it if you feel that the pattern is not optimizing your potential.

As you sit on your chair at the end of the seventh day of induction week, you should take stock of exactly what has been going on. I didn't mention this earlier because I was expecting you pretty much to read the whole book before getting underway, so let me just say at this junction that it would be really good if you would make a journal out of your daily routine. List what you did, when you did it, how you felt during the time, and at the end of the day. Writing what you feel and what you go through is a good way to make it come to the forefront and enhance your resolve for the next day.

Conclusion

Here are a few things that you should have achieved by this point, or, at least, are on the way to achievement over the next few weeks as you make intermittent fasting a way of life. This is, after all, a lifestyle not a course.

At this point:

1. You should have reduced your dependency and habits on scheduled meals.

2. You must have identified and stopped habitual eating.

3. Been able to change your perspective that food is a source of pleasure but, instead, is a source of nutrition and energy.

4. If followed correctly, you should have lost about 8 – 10 pounds of weight in the induction week.

5. You should feel stronger and have a better sense of mind over the body.

6.   You should feel more positive and mentally sharp.

7.   You should come to the realization that all your years of fasting were based on a misconception.

8.   You should realize that you deserve, and are capable of better things.

9.   You know you can do anything.

10.   You should feel better than you have ever felt in your life.

The premise of this book is meant to accomplish two things. First, it is meant to give you a rational understanding of how the body works when it is subjected to fasting, especially intermittent fasting. The second goal of this book is to give you a template to get you started with induction week. I have looked around the web and not many promoters of intermittent fasting understand the value of induction week. However, induction week is as important to a healthy practice of intermittent fasting as stretching and warm-ups are to an athlete.

Intermittent fasting is as much about bringing the mind under control as it is about curbing the intake of food. The alternative to fast or starve one's self in order to lose weight is both unhealthy and unnecessary. Intermittent fasting does it easily, and you can eat what your body asks you to. In fact, that is the whole point. Once you bring your body into the fold and teach it that it can do without junk food, then the body's appetite is the best source of knowing what to eat and when to it. You can even cure ailments and dysfunctions by tuning your diet and listening to what your body wants.

Once you get to that state, then you can be confident that the weight will continue to peel off until you reach your ideal weight. You don't have to listen to what others say should be your ideal shape. Your body will tell you, and you will be that much healthier for it. At that point, you don't have to listen to what others say as you will have the best advice from within you on what to eat, when to eat, and how much to eat. It would be effortless and effective.

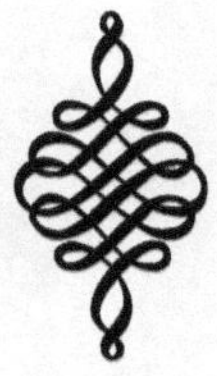

www.ingramcontent.com/pod-product-compliance
Lightning Source LLC
Chambersburg PA
CBHW031322250726
48656CB00005B/1928